Your Journey to a Healthy Life

Great tips and advice for dieting, exercising and making healthy decisions

Kieran Dyer (BSc Hons)

Contents

Introduction

What are the benefits from being healthy?

There are many benefits to becoming healthy, in most cases the reason people choose to diet is to look good achieving that shape that they desire. However, there are way more benefits than just 'looking good'. Firstly, by eating healthy, dieting and exercising you will significantly reduce your risk of certain diseases, like cardiovascular disease, diabetes type II, reduce high blood pressure plus many more. Moreover, through acting out a healthy lifestyle you will also experience a massive boost within your motivation amongst your day to day activities, whilst also increasing your mental well-being, reducing everyday stress levels and become, much happier. Studies have shown that when living a healthy life your sleep pattern improves significantly, perfect setting you up for the day ahead.

Now many people look at exercising and living healthy as kind of a negative, just adding a strain on their way of life. Which at first it may feel a little like this, but there are so many benefits for why you should do this. Living a healthy life can extend your life expectancy, improving your outlook on life, allowing you to really enjoy life to the fullest. There will always be negatives and positives and at first it will be hard to make changes but, after a while you will fall into that daily routine where the strain to eat healthy or exercise will be diminished. When we mention making changes, we don't mean big changes, just certain aspects or things that you know you are doing that can be changed, or prevented to improve your health. As the old saying goes 'small things can make a big difference' and this is true. For example, swapping white bread to wholemeal bread, this small change can make a big difference, brown bread has been shown to be high in fibre, improving blood cholesterol and helps you to feel fuller for longer.

In this eBook you will find that it is divided into three categories, the first being aimed towards dieting tips. Currently there are many diets out there declaring to be the best, helping you lose weight fast etc., etc. This eBook will not mention specific diets, but will help you understand how to monitor your calorie intake and why this is the best way to diet healthily and safely.

Second, the focus will be upon exercising tips such as motivation tips, understanding the physiology behind protein and muscle growth plus much more. This section will help you understand the importance of exercise along with dieting, reason like strengthen your core muscles and the achieving the shape you desire.

The third section will be an understanding of certain diseases that without living heathier, you are at much higher risk of obtaining many common diseases. This section will try to highlight specific factors that people do in their everyday life which could lead to an increase risk of well-known diseases.

We must say that before beginning a lifestyle change for a healthier life it is important that you consult a doctor of your changes you wish to adhere, allowing them to guide you with the safest advice possible.

The reason why this can be important is that doctors can give personal advice suited to your well-being, and body type. In most cases if you are safe and following guidelines then you should be fine, but if you do have any known illnesses that you think may affect your wellbeing then once again seek medical advice.

We do hope that this eBook does help you understand and provide some helpful tips on dieting, health issues and exercise, and that you find it to be helpful. The aim of this eBook is to provide a great insight into all of these areas allowing better understanding helping you to make the best decisions in regards to you own personal health.

As a side note we do ask if you do like this book and you did find it helpful, please help us by writing a review. This would be helpful not only to us, but to those who also decide to purchase the eBook helping others to make the perfect choice. Also, this does allow us to improve our eBooks in the future allowing them to be improved through your mentions to the standard deserved.

Dieting Top Tips

Top 10 tips for losing weight

Losing weight can be very difficult in some cases more mentally than physically. As time goes on the diet becomes much easier as you begin to break out of your old bad habits and learn helpful healthier habits. So here are the top ten tips to make losing weight that little bit easier helping to lead you to a healthier lifestyle.

1. Oops, I forgot to eat breakfast!

A lot of people believe that missing meals will help them lose weight much faster. Well, unfortunately this is not the case, research suggest that those who miss out meals are at higher risk of snacking throughout the day due to hunger cravings. Plus, the body will be starved of vital nutrients for the day ahead. So, don't miss breakfast.

2. Regular meals are important

Eating regular meals actually helps the body burn off calories at a faster rate, whilst as mentioned helps reduce the erg of grabbing that unhealthy snack through that moment of weakness.

Yes, it happens to us all!

Regular meals will allow enough time in between meals to burn off them unwanted calories.

3. Get active and stay active

Exercise is an excellent way to increase your calorie output, plus it has a massive wide array of health benefits, such as strengthening your core muscles and reducing your risk to common illnesses like cardio vascular disease. Being active is best chosen by your interests, exercises you enjoy, which could be joining a gym, running, walking, cycling plus many more.

4. Fruit and veg are key

Many studies have shown fruit and veg to be low in calories and high in fibre, meaning they will help you feel full for longer reducing that craving feeling, but will not have a significant effect on your daily calorie allowance. As a bonus fruit and veg contain the much needed vitamins and minerals.

5. Smaller portion sizes

Reducing the amount you eat at meal times can in some cases be hard, but there are a few tips, like using smaller plate, this will make the meal feel bigger than it is. Also, if you eat out this problem can be combated by ordering a child size meal if possible; and it might save you a bit of money, which is always an added bonus. If ordering children's meals make you feel uncomfortable then just have a small snack meal either as your next meal or the meal before.

6. You can't be tempted if it's not there!

Yes, junk food can be the enemy luring you in when you're at your weakest, okay, a little extreme, but if it's not in the house, then you will not be tempted. Now, I do believe in every diet it is important to treat yourself every now and then, see it as a little reward for doing so well.

But, at the times in your diet when you begin to crave certain junk foods venturing to search the cupboards, by which you tend to realise that if it is not there then you can have it, then you may find an alternative like snacking on fruit.

7. Alcohol

Many people still today think that alcohol doesn't contain any calories. Alcohol does contain calories and in some cases the alcohol content is nearly as high as a piece of chocolate or even a packet of crisps. If you are drinking alcohol try to have a limit and research the calories found in different types of alcohol. Remember most alcoholic beverages are made from a source of carbohydrate or sugar.

8. Eat without any distractions

A recent study has shown that when a person is distracted when eating a meal they are at risk of consuming 40% more calories than if they wasn't distracted. Distraction at meal time, is meant by eating watching television, or on the computer or tablet and the one we all are guilty of browsing on our mobile phones. Just try separating yourself from these distractions when eating and you will feel the difference.

9. Plan your meals ahead

Planning your meals the day before will allow you to keep track of what you are eating, and will give you something to look forward too. Planning your healthy meals will mean that you are at less risk of over indulging, helping you stay on target towards achieving your goal.

10. Weigh each meal accurately

Weighing each meal will help you know your precise calorie intake for each day. This is important, guessing your meal size may prove to be inaccurate leading to an intake of more calories than you anticipated, which will lead to little weight loss and in some cases weight gain.

How to manage a calorie controlled diet

When compared to all of the diets at our disposal, the calorie controlled diet has always been the one to be effective and more importantly, safe. However, saying this, many people have little faith in the calorie controlled diet and always argue that it doesn't work, or some weeks declare that they don't lose any weight at all. In some cases this may be true, but as we all know if you cut corners on a diet, or don't follow a diet correctly, then the results may not be as grateful as you initially hoped.

There are three reason why I personally believe that a calorie controlled diet is the best diet for weight loss, Firstly, because the diet enables a person to learn much more about the importance of all food groups, knowing this allows you to make good choices about how to save on your calorie input whilst still enjoying a great nutritious meal.

Secondly, the diet is focused around consuming a healthy meal, making sure you delve into a meal with vital nutrients, as opposed to leaving major food groups out, which can lead to many health complications.

Thirdly, it is important to lose weight safely, keeping yourself strong throughout diet, and in time any bad eating habits will be swapped for good habits, allowing you to become much healthier.

Food consumption

The recommended daily calorie allowance for a calorie controlled diet for men is 1900Kcal a day, and for women 1400Kcal, these differences are mostly based on the biological makeup of both men and women. These guidance's are suited to the average person of that gender, which may be suited to yourself. But I would advise most people looking to lose weight to make the diet more personal suited to your own BMI and body type. You can do this by searching for a **BMI weight loss calculator.**

I found it to be very helpful.

You must also remember if you are very active or do strength training then your BMI classification will be shown as slightly overweight, which is nothing to worry about, this is normal, if you are strength training you calorie intake will need to be higher than average. The calculator will reveal what your daily calorie intake should be, for example when I did mine it revealed that I should be consuming between 1625-2089 kcal. So, if I for one consumed the normal recommended calorie intake of 2500 kcal then I would be prone to gaining weight, and secondly if I decided to diet on a calorie controlled diet with the recommended 1900kcal, I would probably find myself losing very little weight.

If you do decide to use the calculator then minus off around 200 - 300 kcal revealing your diet calorie allowance, it may be a little trial and error for the first few weeks, but if you do find yourself becoming weak and sluggish just increase your calorie intake slightly until you feel comfortable.

Also, it is very important to plan your daily meals in advance such as, what to have and at what times throughout the day. This will make it much easier to stick to the diet and will give you something to look forward too. It may help by designing a chart with days of the week present, or you may find it easier to plan ahead in a diary.

It is also very important to work out the calorie content of your meal, this can be done with a little research and by weighing your meals. A calorie controlled diet relies on the knowledge of your intake of how many calories you have had a day. Guessing this may lead to inaccurate calorie logging, which in the long run, the diet may not be as effective as you wished. So the more accurate your calorie counting is, the better your result will be. The calories can be calculated either from the packet or you may have to do a little research.

Modern day technology has made it much easier to get our hands on great apps that are at our disposal, searching for apps like meal planners, and daily calorie counters makes it much easier to keep track of your diet, and more importantly stay on track. There are many apps out there; I personally would recommend 'my fitness pal', only because I know people who have used it before and found it very helpful. Try different apps until you find the ones that are suited to your needs.

Remember a diet is the food you consume daily, so adapting habits you don't like will help set you up for a life of health.

Exercise

Exercising when dicting is essential, this will help tone them important core muscles, improving your movement and preventing issues such as back weakness. Plus, exercising will reduce your risk of developing diseases like cardiovascular and diabetes type II. Moreover, exercising will help you develop the desired shape you are looking for. There are a variety of exercises to take part in, some specific for either strength training, or cardio. I believe it is important to take part in regular cardio workouts, which would be accompanied with a little strength training. But it really depends on the type of body you want.

Exercising when dieting can, in some cases, be a little risky if not carried out correctly, therefore on the days which you take part in exercise it is important to monitor you daily calorie input and output, therefore, if your calorie output is high and your calorie input is low then you may want to slightly increase your calorie input. Therefore, I would recommend not having a calorie input lower than 1200 for women, and 1400 for men on normal diet days which would be increased if the exercise was above moderate.

Just remember, that exercise doesn't have to consist of a heavy workouts at the gym, it could easily be a long walk with the dog, or a family cycle; whatever is suited to you!

Weight summary

Ok, stepping on the scales can be; well, scary. But it doesn't need to be. A calorie controlled diet is aimed for you to lose weight slowly and healthily. Losing about 1lb to 2lb a week should be your goal. But on some weeks you may not achieve this, and on other weeks you may lose more than your target weight. This is nothing to be disheartened about, just stick with it and you will succeed.

There are many tips and tricks when coming to weighing yourself, which ever you do is up to you. However, I would recommend weighing yourself on the same day and same time before breakfast every week. Some people find it best to weigh themselves three times and then take the average (add all of the recorded weighing's together and then divide by three). Other tricks consist of making sure you use the same scales every time. Lastly, you may also find that you achieve more by weighing yourself every two weeks rather than every week. However, every week would allow you to keep a more accurate track of your weight.

Remember when dieting it is best to feel comfortable and to try different things to discover what suits you best.

Are carbohydrates and fats really the enemy?

Understanding all food groups is vitally important when adhering to living a healthy lifestyle. Most food groups especially fat and carbohydrates tend to be scrutinised and rendered as unhealthy for you. However, this is not the case, all food groups are required for the body to function and develop healthily. Each category of food plays it role whether it be at the molecular or macro level. However, the balance between the varieties of food groups is required to be balanced, it is only when the diet is unbalance the body tends to develop health complications.

The importance of carbohydrates

The consumption of carbohydrates is commonly related to increasing weight, and is thought to be a leading cause to many health issues. But this is not the case, carbohydrates play many important roles in helping us get through our day to day activities.

Carbohydrates are made up of many glucose molecules bound together in long chains, and when broken down either via cooking, or by our digestive system the chains break apart producing single glucose molecules, (glucose being a sugar).

So what has all of this got to do with our body?

Well, glucose when taken in by our cells is converted to energy. As we know energy plays a key role in our survival. Energy helps us move, grow, fuels our muscle and nervous system and our vital organs.

When consuming carbohydrates it is best to try to stick to the recommended daily allowance which I haven't specified due to this figure being varied in different countries, but it could easily be found with a simple internet search. The main focus is to make sure that your energy intake is either the same or slightly less than your energy output, in other words don't exceed the recommended daily Kcal allowance. Doing so will reduce the risk of any weight gain.

Carbohydrates come in many forms, however selecting wholegrain carbohydrates will allow the body to digest the carbohydrate much slower, releasing the energy gradually, making you feel much fuller for longer, and making it much easier to keep your energy intake below the equilibrium level. Achieving this technique as a lifestyle change will help you stay at a healthy weight and reduce your risk to diseases, such as cardio vascular disease and diabetes. Other tips include introducing more fibre into your diet. Fibre aids and supports digestion, and more importantly helps keeps elevated blood cholesterol in check reducing the risk of arteries becoming blocked.

If you are looking to reduce your carbohydrate intake, it is important to begin cutting out any foods that contain added sugar, whilst also stopping adding sugar to foods. This could be as easy as to not adding sugar to your coffee and cereal. Or buying beverages and foods that are labelled as no added sugar. Although this sounds an obvious change, it is a change that can make such a big difference and is a great starting point when beginning a healthier lifestyle.

Surely fats are not good for you?

All fats are important in our development, for example every cells in our body is made up of phospholipids which is a type of fat, and these phospholipids are bound together with cholesterol, so fats do play a very important role; especially at the micro level. As we are all aware too much of some fats like saturated fats mostly found in foods like butter and lard, pies, cakes and biscuits, fatty cuts of meat, sausages and bacon, and cheese and cream, are not healthy and too much can lead to health complications.

Elevated levels of saturated fat increases blood cholesterol levels, and fat contains 16 calories per gram, which if not used will be stored as fat in adipose tissue as an energy reserve. Increasing your blood cholesterol levels is particularly dangerous and can cause arteries becoming blocked preventing oxygen from reaching areas of the heart or brain, encouraging the onset of many types of diseases like cardiac arrest and stroke.

So what does this mean?

Well, it is important to monitor your fat intake, and more importantly what types of fats you are consuming.

Introduce heart healthy fats into your diet, for example unsaturated fats like polyunsaturated, or even better monounsaturated fats. It is recommended that monounsaturated fats are healthy to use daily. But you must also remember that all unsaturated fats are much healthier for you heart. Also, this doesn't' mean you will need to completely cut out saturated fats from your diet, but it is worth considering significantly reducing your intake. This can be done by cutting the fat off meat or opting to each lean cuts.

Here are some examples of foods that contain goods fats, unsaturated foods will be made up of poly and mono-unsaturated fats, but the fats alone are liquid at room temperature, such as safflower oil, olive oil and corn oil. However, heart healthy fats can be found in many fish foods like salmon, tuna trout and mackerel, presented as omega-3 fatty acid.

Introducing more of these health unsaturated fats more particularly monounsaturated will reduce your risk of obtaining breast cancer, cardio vascular disease and stroke. Plus, other benefits include a reduction in weight loss in some cases targeted more towards belly fat.

Tips to help you stick to a diet

The hardest part about dieting, or changing your diet for healthier options, for many people is sticking with the change in diet. So, I guess the best way to look at dieting is via a lifestyle change, changing your habits, the things you do on an average day, in regards of diet, the foods you are eating. Habits are always difficult to just stop.

It's important to slowly make small changes, making big changes will appear to be much harder adding unneeded stress, which more importantly could prevent you from sticking with the diet. For example, before, we were talking about the calorie controlled diet, personally in my opinion the safest and healthiest way to diet. However, when beginning a calorie controlled diet it is important to slowly reduce calories gradually. For example, if you usually have 2000 calories and want to diet at 1600 calories a day try taking off 200 calories for the first week, and then the second week or two weeks try taking off another 200 calories, and this way it will be much easier to withstand a reduction of calories. It is about making the lifestyle transition much more smother. This process can be done with many aspects, like cutting out chocolate from your diet, gradually cut down and replace with a healthier option, like fruit or crackers.

Along with this technique I have a few more tips to make the change less stressful to help you achieve a much healthier diet.

Set goals and targets

Targets and goals are important when dieting because, they encourage you to be motivated, provide a factor to look forward too, and really allow you to become focused. This is because you really feel that sense of achievement when reaching your goal, which really helps you stay motivated. However, if you do set a target that is harder to achieve, then it may become demotivating if the target is not reached. It is really important to get the balance right. In this respect it may be best to start with small goals, and then build on them gradually, slightly increasing the intensity, therefore the goal is achievable and will lead to better health results.

However, with this in mind, you may always have the same target every day or week. For example, if you are focusing on consuming a certain amount of calories daily, or trying to lose a specific weight. Therefore, it is important to not develop the wrong mind set if you do not achieve your target, so always try to focus on what you have achieved. If you find that you do not constantly achieve your target or goal, then you may be doing something wrong like setting your standards to high. So, either make the goal more achievable for yourself, or try to understand why you didn't achieve the goal and what changes can be made so you can; like if you are trying to reduce your amount of calories, try looking at the foods you are consuming, some foods may fill you up just as much as others but be lower in calories.

Should you plan ahead?

Being organised is extremely helpful when changing your diet. When dieting, some people find it hard and tend to eat little bits throughout the day, which at the end of the day they become tempted to binge, because they haven't eaten much a substantial meal throughout the day. However, if you have a diary or a chart it then allows you to plan your meals ahead, giving you a delicious meal to look forward too, at what time and more importantly knowing the calorie and nutritious content. This will help to keep you from binging, randomly eating, or eating unhealthily. Also, it is good to really understand your diet, this will significantly help you know how the diet may affect your body and what side effects may arise. Many people tend carry out diets that offer a good and fast result, in many cases people tend to either not to foresee the diet through, or more severely they become very ill. Planning healthy meals provides access to good quality food, whilst also achieving the set out daily calorie intake.

The reason why this is important because it interlocks with the step before. If you do set a goal and you diet without a meal plan and lack to monitor what you eating then you may not adhere to that goal you planned ahead, which may again lead to demotivation and a lack of commitment. You will find that planning ahead will allow you to explore other food sources, and eventually you will just eat healthily without a meal plan because it has become a healthy habit.

I deserve a treat!

Okay, this may be a little controversial, but sometimes it's good to indulge in a little treat every now and then. I guess it is best to see it as a reward for your accomplishments, as long as you eating healthy most of the time then it's ok to indulge in a little treat. However, it is important to do this cleverly, for example planning at the end of the week that you're going to have a treat, so you buy a pack of biscuits. Now with the biscuit being insight for a whole week you may have a moment of weakness, if they are not there then you cannot have them, 'out of sight out of mind'. So, I guess what I'm trying to say is that, when you do have a treat do it smaller and kind of spontaneously, in a way that you have subconsciously planned it. This is to prevent the treat from causing temptation and weakness, therefore, helping you and stopping you from indulging unexpectedly.

The size or type of treat is up to you, but try to find out the calorie content. If you do find that you have gone over on your daily allowance don't be too concerned because on some days you may be under. More importantly if you do decide to treat on one day, you should never ever feel disappointed. You must also remember on some days you may have been more active than others days, which will lead to an increase in your calorie outgoings. You will also find that the more you become accompanied with your diet the easier it can be controlled, making it easier for you to choose whether to have a treat or not.

Exercise Top Tips

Top lifestyle tips to achieve the best results from exercising

Exercising, as we know has tremendous benefits on our bodies, whether it be mentally or physically rewarding. But, when working extremely hard at the gym or maybe a long distance run around the local park, you want to make sure that you reek in the best rewards from exercising. Most people find exercising daunting and in some cases don't see the benefit and rewards as fast as they would like to, and tend to just give up. There are so many benefits of exercising both physically and mentally, so it is best to try and stick to exercising making it part of one your weekly activities.

Below are some tips and advice on how to achieve the best from exercising, and more importantly, tips that will help you can stay motivated?

Should I eat before or after exercising?

Many studies have shown that during exercising, the body's metabolic rate increases. This increase is stimulated due to the massive demand for cellular energy to replenish those starving muscles of adenosine triphosphate (ATP).

The recommended time frame for eating after exercise is within a 2 hour window afterwards, but it is advised to wait around 15 minutes before consuming any food.

Most people will grab a quick snack to replace the energy, usually high in protein and carbohydrate, which is fine. However, if you are trying to lose weight, then try eating that healthy balanced meal you had planned. This technique will allow the food ingested to be metabolised much faster, reducing the chances of the food being store as fat.

However, it is advised not to exercise after long periods with food, especially is the exercise is a high endurance routine. This can lead to many health complications. So, plan your exercise routine around your day depending on the type of exercise and any planned meals.

What time is best to exercise?

We have all had the experience, already for your workout, but when you begin you find it tiring, felling a little fatigued, making it hard to engage within the workout. All motivation has been zapped away and you begin to find it difficult to pick up the easiest weight or increase the speed on a tread mill past walking pace, a little dramatic, but you get the point.

In some cases it good to know it may not be your fault. This can be due to the time of the day you work out. Throughout the day our body follows a biological clock, known as the circadian rhythm, which is usually based on the release of specific hormones, such as cortisol, plus many other factors.

These hormones can help provide that spontaneous 'get up and go' feeling. Studies that support this have shown everyone to be different, some do say around 4 pm, whereas some state early morning is best. However, these peaks do happen at various times throughout the day, which is slightly different for each person. So, it is best to try different times throughout the day to find out when you feel you achieve your best performance when exercising. After all, there is nothing worse than not enjoying your workout.

Getting this right will also make the workout a little easier as you will be more mentally ready, wide awake and full of energy. Other factors can play a part also, for example being slightly depressed or stressed after a bad day at work. This will make it hard for you to focus and may cause you to either not try as hard or give up easier.

Should I push myself to workout hard?

I have always said that exercising should be changed to the saying 'getting active'.

Using this term allows people to interpret the term however they please. For example, getting active for someone may be a long country walk 2 or 3 times a week, whereas, to someone else this may mean a daily 5 kilometre run 5 days a week.

The reason why I mention this is that if your exercise routine is more strenuous than you are comfortable with, you are at a higher risk of stopping altogether, by which no benefits of exercising are achieved.

So, it is best when engaging in an exercise to achieve better health, to really think about what exercise you like to challenge yourself with, and what you want to achieve from your exercise routine. Plus, by exercising to a standard that suits your compatibility will help you to gradually increase the intensity when you feel comfortable, and eventually take on new activities.

That is kind of the key here, start off with a type of exercise that you are comfortable with. Doing this will help you make it your weekly routine. Then when the routine is embedded begin either adapting your routine, or increase the intensity gradually which eventually will help you achieve the desired results by which you will be less likely to give up. For example, many people may choose walking as an exercise routine. As you begin, focus on walking a certain route 3-4 times a week. When doing this, track your steps with either an app, or you could just time how long the route takes you. After a few weeks the route will become a normal weekly activity, it is at this stage you can begin to start challenging yourself. Like if you were timing yourself, set a faster target time each week, or you could take longer strides and even make your route longer.

This technique can be used with many types of exercises for example if you are strength training you could either gradually increase your weights, or before you do this, try adding another set to your workout with each exercise. So, if you do 3 sets of 10, try 3 sets of 15 or 4 sets of 10. Doing this will increase the endurance of the workout, make you more mentally strong, and allow your muscles to adopt great fibre repair.

How to stay motivated?

As mentioned throughout staying motivated is important to help keep you on track and achieve a healthier lifestyle. Most people when looking to change their unhealthy habits for healthier ones start off extremely motivated, and after a few weeks begin to struggle. This is because the change is too big making them feel very uncomfortable. This is the same with exercising many people begin don't see the results as fast as they would like and ask themselves is this really worth it?

I must admit with the on goings of everyday life, especially with young children, finding time to exercise can be difficult. It may be a fight at first, but after time it will feel as if it is the norm, leaving you to feel much healthier and much more motivated, not just when exercising but in your everyday life.

Staying motivated is easier when you track your progress, plan ahead and set yourself goals and targets.

Firstly, tracking your progress throughout the weeks or months will allow you to compare from when you began to your current health. The improvement will definitely be enough to help motivate you through those tough times. Tracking your progress can mean recording your heart rate after exercise, physical weight, distance, steps, waist size, weight lifted and many more. There are apps that can help with this, but you can also manually record this, by either designing a chart or keeping track in a diary.

Secondly, organising your week in advance as to the days and time you will exercise tends to put yourself in the mind set of exercising. The idea behind it is that it becomes just another planned activity, increasing the likely hood of completing the routine. This way your exercise will not be spontaneous allowing you to not skip a day, whilst also improving the likely hood of completing the routine on a regular basis. Planning ahead will also enable you to view your schedule allowing you to plan a good time when you know you will be full of energy, like early mornings or straight after a day's work before you go home and relax, but keep in mind the effects of the circadian rhythm, the body's clock, making sure you can commit maximum effort.

Thirdly, and possibly the most important, having a target to reach. Setting a target or various targets can be helpful in two ways. Firstly, by setting target either it be daily, weekly or monthly, will help you to gradually improve your exercise endurance as this allows for the workout to suit your specific needs, and it will add challenge yourself as you improve.

Secondly, beating a target and in some cases not achieving a target set out will encourage you to be more motivated helping you to be focussed and more importantly keep you motivated.

A target can be a variety of things and you can have more than one. For example, using the walking example again. You can set a target to either complete your route by a specific time, or to complete an extra 1000 steps each month. Importantly it is to be remembered that setting a target that measures improvement needs to be small gradual changes that can be achieved with a little extra effort each time, when ready. If the target is set it too hard to achieve, and is not met on regular occasions then this may lead to demotivation which could lead to stopping altogether.

It is important to be in a positive mind set, never view yourself as a failure, even exercising in little stages is better than not at all. However, if your mental wellbeing does change and you begin to feel a little stressed, then try adapting your workout to suit your competence and eventually you will be in a positive mind set to want to work hard again and improve your health and wellbeing.

How Protein Builds Muscle!

Protein is an important part of our diet, and is vital for the maintenance of all body tissues, including muscle. The consumption of protein is broken down into amino acids, required to build a vast array of other proteins and structures.

Becoming ever so popular, are protein supplements, used to gain maximum muscle growth, which is usually consumed following a workout. Although protein can be gained via an introduction of high protein foods to their diet, supplements such as protein shakes or snacks are much more convenient and in some cases can be much cheaper.

So, what is the physiology of muscle growth?

To understand this we need to look at the term muscular hyperplasia!

Muscular hyperplasia is referred to an increase production of myofibrils, mitochondria, sarcoplasmic reticulum and many other organelles. This process occurs as a result of a very forceful, repetitive muscular activity, in other words strength training.

So why increase the production of myofibrils, mitochondria and sarcoplasmic reticulum?

Firstly, myofibrils (also known as the muscle fibre) are the structures that give muscles the striped looked. This is because it is a rod like structure composed of tubular cells called myocytes extending the length of the muscle fibre, housing filaments. Holding these fibres together are proteins called myosin, actin and titin, all which are known as contractile proteins, vital for muscular contraction. The production of these proteins will help bind new muscle fibres and enable contractions with more strength.

Secondly, the mitochondria is a very important organelle for the production of energy and respiration.

Along with calcium (Ca2+) the myosin, actin and titin require phosphorylation. Okay sounds complicated, I will try to explain. The mitochondria produces adenosine triphosphate (you may know it as ATP), which is three phosphate bound to one adenosine molecule. Now, for the activation of myosin, actin and titin they need to steal one phosphate from the ATP. Once bound this will lead to muscular contraction. However, you must remember there are thousands of myosin, actin and titin, meaning this processes occurs many times during each contraction, that's a lot of energy (ATP) required.

Lastly, sarcoplasmic reticulum is an organelle found in the muscle cells (myocytes). The sarcoplasmic reticulum is a vital store for Ca2+, when stimulated upon contraction the sarcoplasmic reticulum will release an out flux of Ca2+ into the cell, which is important to activate myosin, actin and titin via binding just like ATP. Therefore, for new and good muscle fibres to contract, many sarcoplasmic reticulum are required.

All of these protein and structures mentioned, plus other proteins such as messenger proteins and other structural proteins, are why proteins (amino acids) help aid the production of muscle growth. However, among protein, the consumption of vital fats, carbohydrates and vitamins are just as equally important. So, if you do use protein supplements, especially as a meal replacement, ensure that the supplement has all of the vitamins and nutrients required, otherwise you may be wasting your time.

Also, when using supplements it is important to understand any risks involved. For example, long term consumption of high protein has been linked to a person increasing their risk of osteoporosis and certain kidney issues, due to the high blood filtration and pressure. The recommended consumption advised from the Department of Health is to avoid consuming no more than twice the daily recommended intake of protein currently 55.5g for men and 45g for women.

Health Top Tips

Top 5 tips to a achieve a healthier heart

With heart disease effecting millions of people, and becoming more common among 50's and over, looking after your heart seems to be the obvious option. However, the thought of going to the gym, spending all that money and time just seems way too much of a commitment. But, is all of that exercising necessary, well let's find out. Here I have gathered top 5 tips to help focus on achieving a healthier heart.

Blood Pressure:

Monitoring your blood pressure can really be useful in maintaining a healthy heart. The normal range for blood pressure should average around 120/80 mmHg, however, abnormal ranges will consist over 140/90 mmHg, known as high blood pressure or hypertension, when your body is at rest. Constant high blood pressure puts extra strain on the heart forcing the heart to work much harder than it needs to. Therefore, in the long term the heart will strengthen as a muscle, leading to less blood being pumped per beat, causing shortness of breath, nausea, fatigue and much more.

There are simple ways to maintain a low blood pressure mostly by reducing salt intake, eating more fruit and veg, reducing alcohol intake, maintaining a healthy weight and via stopping smoking.

Diet:

Maintaining the perfect BMI can be hard and stressful. In most cases people will try to find a quick fix which usually turns out to be unhealthy and stressful for the body. The best way to think of a diet is to refer to it as what your food intake is currently. Therefore, changing your food intake needs to be a permanent lifestyle choice. So, don't make it too much of a drastic change straight away and slowly ease into the change and adapt as you go along to suit you.

Being overweight is strongly linked to cardiovascular disease. Having extra weight means the body has to supply the extra tissue with blood. So the heart will need to work harder to supply the extra tissue with the requirement of oxygen being carried in the blood.

Also, having a high fat diet can lead to your arteries becoming clogged with fatty substance (atherosclerosis), which in turn leads to narrowing of the coronary arteries. This can easily be overcome by making simple changes to your diet, such as reducing the intake of saturated fat found in foods like butter and lard, pies, cakes and biscuits, fatty cuts of meat, sausages and bacon, and cheese and cream. Also, cut down on snacks between meals especially sugared treats, because excess sugar is converted into a fat store creating adipose tissue.

I know these delicious foods are hard to give up, but you can still have them, as long as you stick to the recommended guidelines for saturated fat which daily is 30g for men and 20g for women. Plus, the saturated fat can be replaced with unsaturated fat eating foods such as, fish and over oily foods, as mention in the previous chapter.

Exercise:

There are many studies conflicting each other, suggesting the recommended amount of exercise and the type of exercise. Exercise has been shown to extend a person's life expectancy by at least 3 years. Whilst some studies have shown that too much vigorous exercise can lead to scaring of the heart tissue, therefore, weakening the heart causing a reduction in blood flow.

So, the subtitle for this paragraph should be called **'Getting active and Staying active'**, this is because going for a cycle, walk at a fast pace, or jogging is more than enough to increase your heart rate. The NHS recommends that a person should complete 150 minutes of weekly physical activity which amounts to 30 minutes on 5 days a week. However, if you are a keen exerciser then only 75 minutes of vigorous activity is recommended.

Remember, this should be a lifestyle change that is kept up and completed on regular occasions. Refer to the previous chapters for more advice.

Alcohol:

I know, unfortunately alcohol can have negative effects on your heart. Alcohol has been linked to many diseases such as, liver disease, cancer, mental illness, plus many more. I guess what we all forget is that alcohol contains calories, in some cases a lot, as shown in the table below.

Drink Calories	(kcal)
Food equivalent	
A standard glass (175ml) of 12% wine	126kcal
1 Cadbury Heroes miniature bar	
A pint of 5% strength beer	215kcal
1 packet of McCoy's salted crisps	
A glass (50ml) of (17%) cream liqueur	118kcal
1 Milky Way bar	
A standard bottle (330ml) of 5% alcopop	
237kcal 3 Lees teacakes	
A double measure (50ml) of 17.5% fortified wine	
65kcal 1 Asda bourbon biscuit	

Adapted from http://www.nhs.uk/Livewell/alcohol/Pages/calories-in-alcohol.aspx.

As mentioned before a high intake of sugar can lead to the production of fatty tissue, especially around the waist line, forcing the heart to work harder.

There are many ways to drink less, such as alternate your drinks with water on a night out, or challenge a friend or family member to cut down with you for support.

Smoking:

Yes, of course smoking. Smoking really does way more harm than good, and I know it is really hard to quit, but stopping smoking reeks with so many benefits, here's why.

Firstly, smoking damages the alveoli in the lungs reducing the surface area for oxygen transfer, forcing the heart to work harder to supply your body with oxygen.

Secondly, nicotine binds to the body's nicotinic receptors which in return leads to a short term rise in blood pressure.

Thirdly, smoking disrupts the clearance of cholesterol (HDL) 'the saturated fat we spoke about earlier' leading to elevated levels of plasma cholesterol, which as mentioned, is strongly linked to cardio-vascular disease.

Once again stopping smoking will show effects even with in the first 40 minutes, and over time will improve your breathing and protect your heart.

Common things you do that can increase cancer risk!

Continuously, the media are always raising concerns over certain exposure or consumptions to certain foods, or lifestyle choices that may lead to specific cancers. Looking at the evidence there are many things that are widely known to be carcinogenic.

However, this maybe a little miss read at times. When something has been labelled carcinogenic, it means that substance is more likely to increase your risk of obtaining a certain types of cancer. Which, in my eyes, is not good, anything that increases your chances of getting cancer should really be left alone.

Which raises the question, what actually does carcinogenic mean?

Well, briefly mentioned before; a substance that is carcinogenic has the ability to manipulate a cell, adapting or changing certain cellular characteristics, allowing the cell to adopt a specific hallmark to encourage the cell to progress unregulated dividing at a much faster rate than other normal cells.

This is mostly due to the carcinogen affecting the DNA, causing mutations which affect certain proteins in the cell, leading to abnormal cellular function. However, in some cases carcinogens can cause abnormal characteristics without causing damage to the DNA. Also, it is usually a chemical or substance that is found in the product or activity being carried out which causes the harm.

There are so many types of cancer causing agents out there however, the four listed seem to be more popular than some others, and are more likely for you to come across in your everyday lives.

Smoking

Starting with the obvious choice. For many years, smoking has been strongly linked to cancer. To begin with, this was a little controversial. This was due to cancer being mostly expressed after many years of consumption (long term use). Due to smoking being extensively studied health care professionals are aware of all the long term and short term negative health effects generated from smoking, cancer being just one.

Smoking has been linked to many cancers. Such as cancers of the lung, oesophagus, larynx, mouth, throat, kidney, bladder, liver, pancreas, stomach, cervix, colon, and rectum, as well as acute myeloid leukaemia.

Yes that many!

This is probably due to there being over 4,000 chemicals found in cigarettes, including 43 known cancer-causing (carcinogenic) compounds and 400 other toxins.

Sunbeds

When I say sunbeds, I really mean UV light exposure, it just so happens that when you are exposed to a significant amount of UV light when using sunbeds obtaining a 'good tan'. There are two types of UV light, these being UVA and UVB, both have been linked to skin cancer, plus premature skin ageing.

This is because UV light has been found to penetrate the skin causing damage to our DNA via dimerization. Dimerization leads to your DNA making bonds that it shouldn't, therefore producing mutations. Much evidence has been carried out in relation to support this link, plus if you look at Australia where the ozone layer is weaker skin cancer tends to be a higher prevalence, than when compare to other countries.

So, if you are a keen tanner, maybe change to applying self-tanning lotion, or at the least you may consider to reduce your exposure time when using sunbeds.

BBQ food

A nice sunny, hot, clear day, (to me) equals BBQ time!

Studies over the last few years have advised that some chemicals when cooking can be carcinogenic.

The theory is that the longer you cook your food, more specifically meat, fish and poultry, the increased chance you have of increasing your risk of cancer.

I know, a bit extreme, but it has been recommended not to overcook your food, you may have noticed especially when BBQing your food, that the edges may become blackened, and it is this that is the carcinogen.

The blackened edges are found to contain heterocyclic amines (HCA). When amino acids and creatine are heated to a high temperature they form HCA which has been found to be carcinogenic. Regular high exposure of HCA have been linked to increasing the risk of cancers of the pancreas, colon and digestive tract.

This doesn't mean you cannot have any more BBQ's, but try to cook the food to a good standard and be aware of HCA, and more importantly, try to reduce your dietary intake of HCAs eliminating regular exposure.

Alcohol

When I think of the negative health benefits of alcohol, for some reason cancer is low on the list. This may be due to some studies showing evidence that a small amount of alcohol will reduce your risk of cancer, this is because alcohol contains antioxidants.

However, alcohol has actually been found to cause 7 types of cancer, including breast, mouth and bowel cancers.

When consuming ethanol (alcohol) our cells convert ethanol to acetaldehyde, which is found to be toxic to our cells damaging DNA and preventing the cells from repairing the damaged DNA. Plus, acetaldehyde has also been found to speed up growth of the hepatocytes, cells in the liver, which may increase the risk to DNA mutations, leading to liver cancer.

So, if possible the advice would be to significantly reduce your exposure of alcohol and just to be on the safe side if you are strong willing, just don't drink it.

I know, easier said than done!

Three ways to reduce your risk of type 2 diabetes

There are two types of diabetes type 1 and type 2. Type 1 is a disease that you are born with and makes up a smaller proportion thought to be around 5-10% of those suffering with the diabetes. Type 2 affecting the larger percentage (90-95%) is acquired later in life. Diabetes is a lifelong illness causing a person's blood sugar level to be raised, leading to many abnormal health complications. Type 2 is either due the beta cells in the pancreas producing too little insulin, or due to insulin receptors being abnormal, rendering the cells inactive to insulin which leads to a reduction in glucose cellular uptake from the blood. In return, the cells cannot produce enough energy due to the lack of glucose.

There are four main risk factors of Type 2 diabetes, these being: age, more common in over 40's or over 25 for south Asians; a strong link with genetics; being at higher risk if a close family member has the disease; the disease is more common with a high BMI either overweight or obese and lastly your ethnic background such as, south Asian, Chinese, African-Caribbean or black African origin.

Everyone's risk to diabetes is different, some may be more susceptible than others. However, regardless of a person's risk they do have some control from acquiring or even slowing down the onset. You may have noticed that most risks cannot be controlled, unless we can stay young or swap our genetics for healthier genes. Maybe someday...........

But, there are things we can do to significantly lower the risk, and take some control of obtaining diabetes, such as:

Monitor your Weight:

As mentioned being overweight or obese increases the chances of obtaining diabetes significantly.

Working at reducing your weight with the advice from the previous chapters will help lower blood glucose levels. Plus, you will also reduce your risk of heart diseases, high blood pressure, and high blood cholesterol levels.

Healthy Eating:

Eating healthy is one of the main important aspects, and most probably the hardest. However, if you get this right, not only will you reduce your high sugar intake, you will also lose weight as an added bonus. Most people find this hard due to the diet intake being due to bad habits. Most unhealthy foods are easily accessible, cheaper and quicker to prepare. However, gradually making slight changes to your dietary intake will help you adapt gracefully. Plus, reading the food labels for sugars and carbohydrates allowing you to not exceed your set maximum daily target. The recommended daily allowance is: Carbohydrates 260 grams and sugars 90 grams, these figures are taken from Public Health England and may differ between genders and/or countries.

Getting active:

When most people think of getting active they imagine themselves joining a gym, spending lots of money, working themselves extremely hard. This is not how it has to be, getting active could mean going for a fast pace walk 3 to 4 times a week, embarking on a regular family bike ride or even joining an active club which interests you, also allowing you will meet others trying to achieve the same goal, As previously mention from the previous chapter on exercise.

There are many tools on the internet to help you with these, just search Food and activity diaries or Meal planners. Using these tools will help you keep track of your progress and help stick to your goals.

Pre-Diabetes:

More and more people are being diagnosed with pre-diabetes, also known as borderline diabetes. This diagnoses does not mean that you are guaranteed to acquire diabetes type 2, or that you have it. However, it is a clear warning sign that you do need to act fast, over wise in the near future you will be diagnosed with Diabetes type II. Pre-diabetes means that your blood sugar levels are higher than normal, but not high enough to be classed as diabetes. Therefore, dietary control and becoming active would be highly recommended, whereby you would once again be at a lower risk.

Before you go

We do hope you found this eBook very helpful.
We would gratefully like to hear your feedback, so we
can improve our next Book.
In the meantime visit Health with a Bite of Science
website to subscribe where you will be kept in form
with our latest releases of our blogs and Books.

www.ingramcontent.com/pod-product-compliance
Lightning Source LLC
Chambersburg PA
CBHW060643290526
45793CB00001B/380